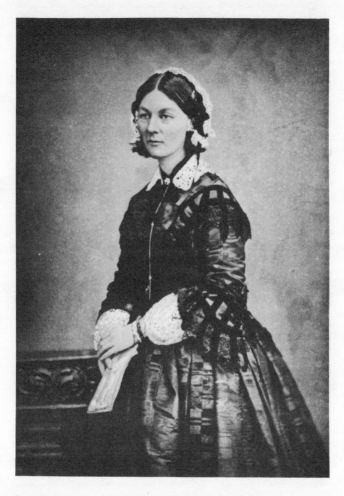

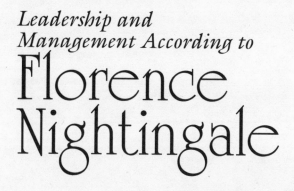

*Leadership and
Management According to*
Florence
Nightingale

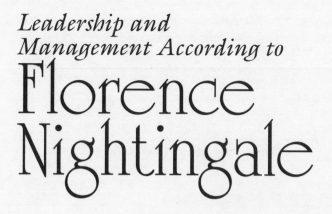

Leadership and Management According to

Florence Nightingale

Beth T. Ulrich, EdD, RN
Vice-President, Patient Services
Northridge Hospital Medical Center
Northridge, California

APPLETON & LANGE
Norwalk, Connecticut

Copyright © 1992 by Appleton & Lange
Simon & Schuster Business and Professional Group

92 93 94 95 96 / 10 9 8 7 6 5 4 3 2 1

Prentice Hall International (UK) Limited, *London*
Prentice Hall of Australia Pty. Limited, *Sydney*
Prentice Hall of Canada Inc., *Toronto*
Prentice Hall Hispanoamericana, S.A., *Mexico*
Prentice Hall of India Private Limited, *New Delhi*
Prentice Hall of Japan, Inc., *Tokyo*
Prentice Hall of Southeast Asia Pte. Ltd., *Singapore*
Editora Prentice Hall do Brasil, Ltda., *Rio de Janeiro*
Prentice Hall, *Englewood Cliffs, New Jersey*

Library of Congress Cataloging-in-Publication Data

Ulrich, Beth Tamplet.
    Leadership and management according to Florence
Nightingale / Beth T. Ulrich.
        p.   cm.
    Includes bibliographical references.
    ISBN 0-8385-5642-6
    1. Nursing services—Administration.   2. Leadership.
  3. Nightingale, Florence, 1820–1910—Views on management.
  4. Nightingale, Florence, 1820–1910—Views on leadership.
  I. Title.
  RT89.U47   1992
  362.1'73'068—dc20   92-6793
                                                             CIP

Executive Editor: William Brottmiller
Senior Editor: Barbara Norwitz
Production Editors: Sandra Huggard, Sasha Kintzler
Designers: Janice Barsevich, Michael Kelly

PRINTED IN THE UNITED STATES OF AMERICA

*To Florence, who first carried the lamp,
and my colleagues,
who continue to light the way.*

Contents

Overview 1

Change 11

Communication 15

Hospitals 23

Leadership 39

Negotiation 61

Organizational Structure 67

Personnel Issues 75

Physicians 85

Power 93

Time Management 103

A Final Note From Florence 111

References 113

Bibliography 125

Overview

At some point in nursing school, each of us was introduced to Florence Nightingale, the lady with the lamp. We were told that she cared for soldiers in the Crimea and started one of the first real schools of nursing, as well as having penned a nursing text.

As my years in nursing have passed, I've occasionally looked to Florence for words of wisdom, especially when giving speeches. Only recently did I become interested in her as a role model for patient care administrators. Her numerous writings and experiences are valuable learning tools both for what to do to be a successful administrator as well as sometimes teaching us what not to do.

When most of us "met" Florence, we never realized what phenomenal organizational and administrative skills she possessed. Further, we never appreciated the conditions under which she exhibited her skills.

Background. Florence Nightingale was born on May 12, 1820, and reared as the elder daughter of affluent British parents. Like many of us, she began early in life "nursing" her sick dolls. She was also said to have a special touch with injured animals. Her parents saw it all as a passing fancy. Florence saw it as the beginning of a life of service. As she grew into a woman, she found excuse after excuse to visit hospitals throughout Europe, learning what she could from each until, finally, she felt ready to begin her career.

Florence's first position, taken in August, 1853, at age thirty-three, was that of Resident Lady Superintendent of the Invalid Gentlewomen's Institution on Upper Harley Street in London. It was a small charity hospital that was very run down and poorly managed. Florence moved quickly to make major changes in the manner in which care was delivered, restricting how long the patients could stay, and writing the institution's first public advertisement. Her people management skills, however, had not yet been well developed, and she experienced almost a one hundred percent turnover in her staff in the first three months. Not all of the turn-over was bad for the institution, but nei-ther was it all planned.

In October, 1854, having, in her estimate at least, accomplished all she could at Up-per Harley Street, Florence saw a new challenge in answering the call to care for the soldiers in the Crimea, where Britain, France, and Turkey were at war with Rus-sia. She and her nurses arrived by boat in Scutari in the Crimea on November 4, 1854. Before leaving Britain, Florence had been told that she would be in charge of nursing and that she would have all the supplies she needed. On the contrary, when Florence and her nurses arrived in Scutari, she found scarce supplies and a decidedly unwelcoming atmosphere. She was in charge of several hospitals in Scu-tari and Balaclava. The main hospital, lo-cated in Scutari, was a dilapidated quadrangle building, one-quarter mile on each side, housing four miles of hospital beds, and filled with pests and unsanitary conditions. An additional problem was the overtly cold and unwelcoming attitude of the physician staff who saw the nurses as only getting in the way. Rather than bully her way in, Florence chose a more moderate and calculated approach. With a belief that dirt was related to disease, she quickly set the nurses to cleaning the hospital—having to get rid of not only filth and pests, but also heaps of body parts that had been amputated from the soldiers. The next step was to clothe and feed the soldiers, which she also accomplished, all the while instructing her nurses not to deliver nursing care until the physicians approved it. The turning point came in only a few days when, as result of 50,000 Russians attacking 8,000 British at the Battle of Inkerman, 2,500 British casualties descended on the Barrack Hospital at Scutari. Suddenly, the doctors welcomed the nurses. As if things were not bad enough with only forty nurses and almost 2,500 patients, a hurricane hit Scutari the following week, sinking the ship in Balaclava Harbor that was bringing in medical supplies, clothing, food, and military equipment. If Florence had not learned how to creatively procure and manage resources before, she certainly had to quickly develop those skills. Over the next few months, she did just that, even expanding the services she and the nurses provided. Her position in the Crimea became, in many ways, like that of the patient care administrator of today. As F.B. Smith, one of her biographers, noted, "she herself did little actual nursing at the hospitals. By day, she negotiated with the doctors, drove orderlies, and inspected stores, the nurses' work, and hospital maintenance. By night, she broke her own rules about walking the wards alone . . . inspecting the patients and wards, noting the dying" (p. 40).

While many nurses know only of Florence's nursing in the Crimea, her subsequent penning of *Notes on Nursing*, and her being responsible for opening the St. Thomas School of Nursing, these were only the mere beginnings of her long career in health care. After returning home from the Crimea, Florence turned her energies towards restructuring the health care system of the British Army and establishing a Royal Sanitary Commission for India. For many years after the School of Nursing was opened at St. Thomas in 1860, she reviewed the written work of all of the students, wrote critiques of their papers, and invited the most promising students to have tea with her periodically. She became involved in hospital design projects in a number of countries, and tried valiantly to persuade the health care authorities of the value statistics could have in improving health care. She became a prolific author, writing some 200 books, articles, and reports as well as over 12,000 letters. Until well into her eighties, she remained active, mostly playing the behind-the-scenes role she enjoyed, but maintaining her power throughout. This is all the more impressive when one realizes that, after age thirty-nine, she spent most of her life in bed. She suffered from a variety of illnesses that kept her homebound, some as a result of her own bout with the Crimean fever, and some, her biographers speculate, as a result of her desire to control her life and have other people work on her schedule. When she died on August 13, 1910 at the age of ninety, Florence had outlived her immediate family and most of her colleagues.

Why do I call her "Florence?" By now, you have already noticed that I generally refer to Florence Nightingale as "Florence." Most authors call her "Miss Nightingale" in their works, making her seem (to me, anyway) formal and unreachable. The more I read in preparing this book, the more I began to think of Florence as a colleague—a fellow patient care administrator who went through many of the same highs and lows you and I go through every day. She wasn't perfect. She too made mistakes. But she learned from those mistakes. Since "Florence" was the formal version of her first name (her friends called her "Flo,"), and since she herself seemed to find joy in nicknaming her acquaintances, I don't think she would mind her colleagues of this century calling her "Florence."

Leadership and Management According to Florence. After reviewing a large amount of Florence's correspondence as well as much of the material written about her, I have compiled this book as an interpretation of Florence's principles of management and leadership. It is my sincere hope that you are as inspired by her words as I have been and as awed by how much she knew over a hundred years ago that we can still learn from today.

Editorial Notes: As much as possible, the punctuation and spelling included in this book are as they appear in the original documents; however, in some cases, there are multiple "originals" of the same letter. Florence had a habit of making and keeping copies of her letters to others, and the copies were not always exactly like the original. Her direct quotes are always presented in *italics*. Also, the author would ask the indulgence of male nurses in understanding that Florence meant no sexism by calling nurses women. One only has to read her comments on sexism to know that she was only writing about things as they were in her time and not as she would have expected them to be in the future.

For us who Nurse, our Nursing is a thing, which, unless in it we are making progress every year, every month, every week, take my word for it, we are going back.

Change

No system can endure that does not march. Are we walking to the future or to the past? Are we progressing or are we stereotyping? We remember that we have scarcely crossed the threshold of uncivilized civilization in nursing: there is still so much to do. Don't let us stereotype mediocrity. We are still on the threshold of nursing.[1]

One of Florence's biographers, F. B. Smith, has described the talents that made her a successful change agent:

1. She found and enlisted people who had the skills to define the problems and formulate the solutions.
2. Once she had been briefed on the problems and potential solutions, she could state the case clearly and could marshal a large amount of personal force and persistence in seeing the change through.

3. She was extremely astute to who had power in a given situation and whose ambitions could be used in aligning their power with hers.
4. She held steadfast in the belief that whatever change she wanted to make was practically and morally right.

In Florence's own mind, the world needed people who were willing to create change:

There are two classes of people in the world—those who take the best and enjoy it and those who wish for something better and try to create it. The world needs the appreciation of the first and the discontent of the second.[2]

About change, she also wrote in one of her annual addresses to the probationers and nurses of the St. Thomas School, given in May, 1872:

To be a good nurse, one must be a good woman, or one is nothing but a tinkling bell. To be a good woman at all, one must be an improving woman, for stagnent waters sooner or later, and stagnent air, as we know ourselves, always grow corrupt and unfit for use.[3]

For us who Nurse, our Nursing is a thing, which, unless in it we are making <u>progress</u> every year, every month, every week, take my word for it, we are going <u>back</u>.[4]

Part of Florence's success as a change agent was a result of her ability to be flexible. Her words on the subject are the kind of common sense thoughts that seem simple, but are so easily forgotten in the often chaotic world of health care.

o not be fettered by too many rules at first. Try different things and see what answers best.[5]

Look for the ideal, but put it into the actual.[6]

Everything which succeeds is not the production of a scheme, of rules and regulations made beforehand, but of a mind observing and adapting itself to wants and events.[7]

*Let us each & all realizing
the importance of our influence
on others—stand shoulder
to shoulder—& not alone,
in good cause.*

Communication

The most obvious lesson Florence teaches us about communication is to do it. In her lifetime, she wrote over 200 books, articles, and reports, and over 12,000 letters. Often her letters include a thank-you or a positive personal statement about some action the letter recipient has taken. She always found time to write, even when she was busiest. Time and again, relationships built or solidified through her written correspondence proved to be useful when Florence wanted to accomplish something. As Monteiro said so well in 1972, "The power of her pen was felt throughout the world" (p. xvii).

Zachary Cope, in his work *Florence Nightingale and the Doctors*, has noted that Florence had two distinct personalities that came through especially in her writing. Her public personality, the one seen in her official communications, was discreet, diplomatic, and tactful, anxious to obtain information and careful not to arouse animosities. Her private personality, which she let her close friends, family, and trusted confidants see, was open and uninhibited. In fact, she often requested that the recipients either burn her private correspondence or return it to her. On some occasions, especially with Sir Harry Verney with whom she has both a public relationship and later a private one as his sister-in-law, she would write two letters to the same person about the same topic. The thoughts in one of the letters could be used publicly while whose in the other she expected to remain private.

In her position as the Resident Lady Superintendent of the Invalid Gentlewomen's Institution at Upper Harley Street, Florence initiated quarterly written communications to the Ladies' Committee to whom she reported. For the first time, the governing committee was given regularly, in writing, information on patient census and disposition as well as information on operations and finances.

With regard to verbal communication, she admitted to her friend and mentor Sidney Herbert (December 25, 1854) that she was not always the calm, serene person she was often pictured to be. In describing her reaction to some of the physician and provision problems she encountered in Scutari, she said:

>Such a tempest has been brewed in this little pint-pot as you could have no idea of. But I, like the ass, have put on the lion's skin, and when once I have done that, (poor me, who never affronted anyone before), I can bray so loud that I shall be heard, I am afraid, as far as England.
>
>However, this is no place for lions & as for asses, we have enough.[8]

Florence had a habit of writing notes to herself as well as to others. In one such note written in 1857, she summarized one of the reasons she thought communication was so important.

>If we are permitted to finish the work which He gave us to do, it matters little how much we suffer doing it. In fact, the suffering is part of the work

& contingent upon the time or period of the world at which we were sent into it to do its work. But surely, it is also part of the work to tell the world what we have suffered & how we have been hindered, in order that the world may be able to spare others. To act otherwise is to treat the world as an incorrigible child which cannot *listen or as a criminal which will* not *listen to right.*[9]

Florence learned quickly the art of communicating with groups, often in committees. In a letter to her father some three months after beginning her work at Upper Harley Street (December 3, 1853), Florence described her committee work:

hen I *entered the service here, I determined that, happen what would, I* never *would intrigue among the Comtee. Now I perceive that I do all my business by intrigue. I propose in private to A, B, or C the resolution I think A, B, or C most capable of carrying in Committee, and then leave it to them—and I always win.*[10]

Further in the same letter, she talks about how she got five resolutions passed, but also about the potential for her plan to have backfired.

All these I proposed and carried in Committee without telling them that they came from me and not from the medical men; and then, and not until then, I showed them to the medical men, without telling them they were already passed in Committee. It was a bold stroke but success is said to make an insurrection into a revolution. The medical men have had two meetings upon them and approved them all and thought they were their own. And I came off with flying colours, no one suspecting my intrigue, which of course would ruin me if it were known, as there is much jealousy in the Committee of one another, and among the medical men of one another.[11]

Despite her early manipulating of committees, Florence soon learned the importance of teamwork. In her 1872 address to the nurses and students at St. Thomas, she said:

> The very essence of all good organisation is that every body should do her (or his) own work in such a way as to help and not hinder every one else's work.[12]

In another of her addresses in 1881, she issued a challenge:

> We all see how much easier it is to sink to the level of the low, than to rise to the level of the high: but dear friends all, we know how soldiers were taught to fight in the old times against desperate odds: standing shoulder to shoulder & back to back. Let us each & all realizing the importance of our influence on others—stand shoulder to shoulder—& not alone, in good cause.[13]

It may seem a strange principle to
enunciate as the very first requirement
in a Hospital that
it should do the sick no harm.
It is quite necessary nevertheless
to lay down such a principle.

Hospitals

Florence was clear on her feelings about the use of hospitals as early as in her second quarterly report to the Ladies' Committee at Upper Harley Street (February 20, 1854).

 Hospital is *good for the seriously ill alone—otherwise it becomes a lodging-house where the nervous become more nervous, the foolish more foolish, the idle & selfish more selfish & idle.*[14]

She subsequently set rules in place that prohibited any patient from staying longer than two months unless she was dying. Florence's reasoning was clear in a letter she wrote to her father in 1854.

 ll *must go at the end of 2 months, except those dying. Otherwise, there is no incentive to get well.*[15]

In *Notes on Hospitals* (1863), she further said that when patients do go to a hospital, they should get in and out as quickly as possible.

t is a rule without any exception that no patient ought ever to stay a day longer in a hospital than is absolutely essential for medical or surgical treatment.[16]

Her reasoning for making the time in a hospital as short as possible was seen in the preface of the same book.

t may seem a strange principle to enunciate as the very first requirement in a Hospital that it should do the sick no harm. It is quite necessary nevertheless to lay down such a principle, because the actual mortality in hospitals, especially in those of large crowded cities, is very much higher than any calculation founded on the mortality of the same class of patient treated <u>out</u> of hospitals would lead us to expect.[17]

Florence went so far as to say, in her *Introductory Notes on Lying-In Institutions* (1871), that birthing (a well process) should be separated from illness.

ince lying-in is not an illness, and lying-in cases are not <u>sick</u> cases, it would be well, as already said, to get rid of the word 'hospital' altogether, and never use the word in juxtaposition with lying-in women, as lying-in women should never be in juxtaposition with any infirmary cases.[18]

Finally, in 1893, in a paper she wrote for a congress (held with the World's Fair in Chicago) on nursing, hospitals, and dispensaries, she expressed hope for the future.

n the future, which I shall not see, for I am old, may a better way be opened! May the methods by which every infant, every human being, will have the best chance of health, the methods by which every sick person will have the best *chance of recovery, be learned and practiced! Hospitals are only an intermediate stage of civilization, never intended, at all events, to take the whole sick population.*[19]

Florence became involved in hospital design and construction, and, in the case of St. Thomas Hospital in 1860, in developing what today we would call a market analysis. The Railway Company wanted part of the hospital's land to extend railway services. Some hospital officials wanted the railway company to buy all of the hospital's land or none. If they bought all, the hospital would then be rebuilt on a new site. Other hospital officials thought that the Railway Company should be able to just buy the part of the hospital's land it needed; portions of the hospital on the land bought would then be rebuilt on other adjacent hospital land. Florence's opinion was sought and she proceeded to perform a market analysis. She gathered and analyzed data on the origin (by location) of the hospital's patients, determining how many patients would be affected if the hospital were moved to various potential sites. The results showed that many fewer patients than had been suspected would have to travel longer distances to reach the hospital. This inconvenience, she proposed, would be offset by the advantages of a new facility on a new site. Given her data, the officials agreed.

In *Notes on Hospitals*, Florence was specific about her view on hospital architects.

Effectual and easy supervision is essential to proper care and nursing. And, as everybody knows, a patient may often be saved by careful nursing when everything else will fail. It is at this point that the hospital architect may either facilitate or prevent recovery to the extent to which his plan renders nursing easy, or the reverse.[20]

Further in the same book, she talks about hospital design aspects many of which appear as applicable today as when her book was written in 1863.

It is a fundamental principle that the pavillions, whether single or *double, should contain nothing but the sick and the offices immediately required for the ward. Everything else, board rooms, chapels, quarters for officers and servants, except for the head nurse or nurses of each ward, stores, kitchens, laundries, should be placed in a separate building or buildings. It would be better even that convalescent rooms, where it is determined that there should be such rooms, should be out of the main building, but accessible under cover; for the obvious reason that convalescents require change of air which cannot be obtained under any circumstances in a hospital.*[21]

Florence was adamant that an important part of hospital and health care administration was the effective use of data and statistics. For a person not trained formally in the use of such tools, she certainly knew how to use both to the advantage of her causes. She believed that statistics were the basis for exact social laws and could predict the moral consequences to various actions.

In her *Notes on Matters Affecting the Health, Efficiency and Hospital Administration of the British Army*, she filled over 830 pages with her recommendations, many of which she reinforced with statistical tables and exploding piecharts. Smith (1982) notes that her use of the word "efficiency" in the title of this book represents one of the first times the word was used in the modern sense. Florence was again ahead of her time, as "efficiency" did not become a part of the official British military vocabulary until 1864.

Much of this book concerned sanitary reform, a central theme of many of her patient and army personnel proposals. It was a theme she knew would garner support from many quarters and one she used to the fullest.

Florence also foresaw the need for statistically comparing outcome data both by treatments and interventions, and by hospitals. Over a hundred years before the United States Health Care Finance Administration was beginning to publish comparative data, Florence was proposing such a system in detail!

In 1860, Florence presented a proposal for a uniform hospital statistical system to the International Statistical Congress in London. With regard to what we now call utilization review and resource allocation, she suggested that statistics could be used effectively.

They would enable us to ascertain . . . what diseases and ages press most heavily on the resources of particular hospitals. For example, it was found that a very large proportion of the limited finances of one hospital was swallowed up by one preventable disease— Rheumatism—to the exclusion of many important cases or other diseases from the benefits of hospital treatment.[22]

She saw a use for statistics to evaluate the quality of medical care and proposed forms for that purpose.

They [the proposed forms] would enable the mortality in hospitals, and also the mortality from particular diseases, injuries, and operations, to be ascertained with accuracy; and these facts, *together with the duration of cases, would enable the value of particular methods of treatment and of special operations to be brought to statistical proof.*[23]

In the same presentation, Florence also suggested that statistics could be used to look at cost effectiveness and cost benefit analyses.

hese statistics would show subscribers how their money was being spent, what amount of good was really being done with it, or whether the money was doing mischief rather than good . . . They would enable us to ascertain the mortality in different hospitals, as well as from different diseases and injuries at the same and different ages, the relative frequency of different diseases and injuries among the classes which enter hospitals in different countries, and in different districts of the same country. They could enable us to ascertain how much of each year of life is wasted by illness.[24]

The Congress communicated her proposals to the governments of the countries represented at the Congress. Unfortunately, the forms were too complicated and were quickly abandoned by the hospital officers. One wonders what these same hospital officers would think of the forms of today.

Undaunted, Florence continued to pursue her cause. In *Notes on Hospitals*, published in 1863, she further developed her effort of collecting and effectively using comparative data, as well as introducing concepts that we would much later know as comorbidities, length of stay, and outcome criteria. In addition, she could have taught the data gatherers of today a thing or two about how the system could be gamed.

It is sometimes asserted that there is no such striking difference in the mortality of different hospitals as one would be led to infer from their great apparent difference in sanitary condition. There is, undoubtably, some difficulty in arriving at correct statistical comparison to exhibit this. For, in the first place, different hospitals receive very different proportions of the same class of diseases. The ages in one hospital may differ considerably from the ages in another and the state of the cases on admission may differ very much in each hospital. These elements affect considerably the results of treatment, altogether apart from the sanitary state of hospitals.

. . . In the next place, accurate hospital statistics are much more rare than is generally imagined, and at best they only give the mortality which has taken place in the hospitals, and take no cognizance of those cases which are discharged in a hopeless condition, to die immediately afterwards, a practice which is followed to a much greater extent by some hospitals than others.

We have known incurable cases discharged from one hospital, to which the deaths ought to have been accounted, and received into another hospital, to die there in a day or two after admission, thereby lowering the mortality rate of the first at the expense of the second.

The sanitary state of any hospital ought not, however, to be inferred solely from the greater or less mortality. If the function of a hospital were to kill the sick, statistical comparisons of this nature would be admissable. As, however, its proper function is to restore the sick to health as speedily as possible, the elements which really give information as to whether this is done or not, are those which show the proportion of sick restored to health, and the average time which has been required for this object; a hospital which restored all its sick to health after an average of six months' treatment could not be considered as by any means so healthy as a hospital which returned all its sick recovered in as many weeks. The proportion of recoveries, the proportion of deaths, and the average time in hospital, must all be taken into account in discussions of this nature, as well as the character of the cases and the proportion of different ages among the sick; and this brings me to the great importance of

correct hospital statistics as an essential
element of hospital administration.[25]

Further in the same book, Florence suggested that statistics could be used to look
at cost effectiveness and cost or outcome
benefit analysis.

I *am fain to sum up with an urgent
appeal for adopting this or some
uniform system of publishing the
statistical records of hospitals. There is a
growing conviction that in all hospitals,
even in those which are best conducted,
there is a great and unnecessary waste of
life; and that, as a general rule, the poor
would recover better in their own miserable
dwellings if they had proper medical and
surgical aid, and efficient nursing, than
they do under more refined treatment in
hospitals. But few have had so sad or so
large an experience as I have had to lead
them to this conviction. It is imperative
that this impression should be either
dissipated or confirmed.*

In attempting to arrive at the truth, I

have applied everywhere for information, but in scarcely an instance have I been able to obtain hospital records fit for any purposes of comparison. If they could be obtained, they would enable us to decide many other questions besides the ones alluded to. They would show subscribers how their money was being spent, what amount of good was really being done with it, or whether the money was not doing mischief rather than good: they would tell us the exact sanitary state of every hospital and of every ward in it, where to seek for causes of insalubrity and their nature; and, if wisely used, these improved statistics would tell us more of the relative value of particular operations and modes of treatment than we have means of ascertaining at present. They would enable us, besides, to ascertain the influence of the hospital with its numerous diseased inmates, its overcrowded and possible ill-vented wards, its bad site, bad drainings, impure water, and want of cleanliness—or the reverse of all these—upon the general course of

*operations and diseases passing through its
wards; and the truth thus ascertained
would enable us to save life and suffering,
and to improve the treatment and
management of the sick and maimed
poor.*[26]

Finally, regarding hospitals, Florence of-
fered those of us who work in them a
warning in an address to the students and
nurses of St. Thomas given on May 23,
1873:

*he world, more especially the
Hospital world, is in such a hurry,
is moving so fast, that it is too easy to
slide into bad habits before we are aware.*[27]

Let who ever is in charge keep this simple question in her head (<u>not</u>, how can I always do this right thing myself, but) how can I provide for this right thing to always be done?

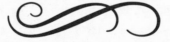

Leadership

There is little doubt that Florence was a leader, not only in nursing, but in many aspects of the health care system. Her demeanor of calm dignity is said to have influenced everyone with whom she came in contact. She was especially effective in subtlely leading men in authority in an age when women were rarely heard. Tooley (1910) attributes Florence's influence over these men to her not being dictatorial or aggressive, but rather to her having possessed judgment that inspired confidence and knowledge that compelled respect and attention.

Another of her biographers, F. B. Smith (1982) saw two great strengths in Florence which accounted for her success as a reformer: "she defined issues and goals . . . in the pursuit of which she never faltered," and "she had also an extraordinarily rich and firm imaginative grasp of the relations between individuals and the siting and working of things and human beings' relation to them" (p. 12).

As we will see throughout this chapter, Florence had a set of values and principles on which she believed nursing and the leadership of nursing should be based. In an address to the nurses and students of St. Thomas in 1875, she described her belief thusly.

What is our needful thing? To have high principles at the bottom of all. Without this, without having laid our foundation, there is small use in building up our details. That is as if you were to try to nurse without eyes or hands ... If your foundation is laid in shifting sand, you may build your house, but it will tumble down.[28]

Early on, Florence found out about the aspect of leadership later referred to as "the buck stops here." When she got the rule enacted at Upper Harley Street prohibiting patients from staying longer than two months, she had no idea that she would be the one to enforce it. As she wrote to her father in 1854:

y Committee have not the courage to discharge a single case. <u>They</u> say the Medical Men must do it. The Medical Men say <u>they</u> won't, although the cases they say <u>must</u> be discharged. And I <u>always</u> have to do it, as the stop gap on all occasions.[29]

In her writings, especially *Notes on Nursing*, Florence often talks about what it takes to be a leader.

ll the results of good nursing, as detailed in these notes, may be spoiled or utterly negatived by one defect, viz.: in petty management, or, in other words, by not knowing how to manage that what you do when you are there, shall be done when you are not there. The most devoted friend or nurse cannot always be <u>there</u>. Nor is it desirable that she should. And she may give up her health, all her other duties, and yet, for want of a little management, be not one-half as efficient as another who is not

*one-half so devoted, but who has that art
of multiplying herself—that is to say, the
patient of the first will not really be so
well cared for as the patient of the second.*

*It is as impossible in a book to teach a
person in charge of sick people how to
<u>manage</u>, as it is to teach her how to
nurse. Circumstances must vary with each
different case. But it is possible to press
upon her to think for herself: Now what
does happen during my absence? I am
obliged to be away on Tuesday. But fresh
air, or punctuality is not less important to
my patient on Tuesday than it was on
Monday.*[30]

As an example, she responds to the case
of a person in charge not being on duty
when an event occurred:

*The person in charge was quite right
not to be '<u>there</u>,' he was called
away for quite sufficient reason, or he was
away for a daily recurring and
unavoidable cause: yet no provision was
made to supply his absence. The fault was*

not in his `*being away*,' but in there
being no management to supplement his
`*being away*.' When the sun is under total
eclipse or during his nightly absence, we
light candles. But it would seem as if it
did not occur to us that we must also
supplement the person in charge of sick or
of children, whether under an occasional
eclipse or during a regular absence.[31]

Other notes on being in charge include:

Let who ever is in charge keep this
simple question in her head (not,
how can I always do this right thing
myself, but) how can I provide for this
right thing to always be done?

Then, when anything wrong has
actually happened in consequence of her
absence, which absence we will suppose to
have been quite right, let her question still
be (not, how can I provide against any
more of such absences? which is neither
possible or desireable, but,) how can I
provide against any thing wrong arising
out of my absence?[32]

... How *few men, or even women, understand, either in great or in little things, what it is the being "in charge"*—I mean, *know how to carry out a "charge." From the most colossal calamities, down to the most trifling accidents, results are often traced (or rather not traced) to such want of some one "in charge" or of his knowing how to be "in charge."*[33]

To be 'in charge' *is certainly not only to carry out the proper measures yourself but to see that every one else does so too; to see that no one either wilfully or ignorantly thwarts or prevents such measures. It is neither to do everything yourself nor to appoint a number of people to each duty, but to ensure that each does that duty to which he is appointed.*[34]

Again, *people who are in charge often seem to have a pride in feeling that they will be 'missed,' that no one can understand or carry on their arrangements, their system, books,*

accounts, & etc. but themselves. It seems
to me that the pride is rather in carrying
on a system, in keeping stores, closets,
books, accounts, &c., so that any body
can understand and carry them on—so
that, in case of absence or illness, one can
deliver every thing up to others and know
that all will go on as usual, and that one
shall never be missed.[35]

Florence also stated in *Notes on Nursing*
that she believed that the person in charge
of any building should:

Think it necessary to visit every hole
and corner of it every day. How
can she expect those who are under her to
be more careful to maintain her house in
a healthy condition than she who is in
charge of it? . . . Don't imagine that if
you, who are in charge, don't look to all
these things yourself, those under you will
be more careful than you.

But again, to look at all these things
yourself does not mean to do them
yourself . . . If you do it, it is by so
much the better, certainly, than if it were

not done at all. But can you not insure
that it is done when not done by
yourself? Can you insure that it is not
undone when your back is turned? This is
what being 'in charge' means. And a very
important meaning it is, too. The former
only implies that just what you can do
with your own hands is done. The latter
that what ought to be done is always
done.[36]

In her 1867 annual address to the students and nurses of St. Thomas, she
talked about authority in depth.

What are the qualities which give us
authority, which enable us to
exercise some charge or control over others
with "authority?" It is not the charge or
position itself, for we often see persons in
a position of authority, who have no
authority at all; and on the other hand
we sometimes see persons in the very
humblest position who exercise a great
influence or authority on all around them.
The very first element for having control

over others is, of course, to have control over oneself. If I cannot take charge of myself, I cannot take charge or others. The next, perhaps, is—not to try to 'seem' anything, but to <u>be</u> what we would seem.

A person in charge must be felt more than she is heard—not more than she is felt. She must fulfil her charge without noisy disputes, by the silent power of a consistent life, in which there is no <u>seeming</u>, and no hiding, but plenty of discretion. She must exercise authority without seeming to exercise it.

A person, but more especially a woman, in charge must have a quieter and more impartial mind than those under her, in order to influence them by the best part of them and not by the worst.

. . . We must not give an order, much less a reproof, without being fully acquainted with both sides of the case. Else, having scolded wrongfully, we look rather foolish.

The person in charge every one must see to be just and candid, looking at both sides, not moved by entreaties or, by likes *and dislikes, but only by justice; and always reasonable, remembering and not forgetting the wants of those of whom she is in charge.*

She must have a keen though generous insight into the characters of those she has to control. They must know that she <u>cares</u> for them even while she is checking them; or rather that she checks them <u>because</u> she cares for them.[37]

Further in the same address, she discussed the improper use of being in an authoritative position.

I have been in positions of authority myself and have always tried to remember that to use such an advantage inconsiderately is—cowardly. To be sharp upon them is worse in me than in them to be sharp upon me. No one can trample upon others and govern them. To win them is half, I might say the whole, secret of "having charge." If you find your way to their hearts, you may do what you like with them; and that authority is

*the most complete which is least perceived
or asserted.*[38]

She believed that being a leader sometimes meant taking action regardless of
what might occur. In one case, while she
was in the Crimea, patients were desper-
ately hungry and the nourishments they
needed were stored in a nearby warehouse. The "rule" was that the nourishments could not be released until after an
official inspection. Florence first tried to
get the inspection done. She had no success. Then she asked the purveyor to re-
lease the nourishments without an
inspection. She still had no success. Finally, she took two soldiers with her, went
to the warehouse, opened the doors, and
took the supplies the patients needed!

Florence clearly saw the struggles of
leadership. She wrote to her family from
Scutari in 1854:

*ould anyone but know the
difficulties and heart-sinkings of
command, the constant temptation to
throw it up . . .*[39]

Regardless of what actions were required of a leader, Florence felt that she and others had to take responsibility for their own actions and not to make excuses. In a letter to H. Bonham Carter in 1861, she said:

 have had a larger responsibility of human lives than ever man or woman had before. And I attribute my success to this:——I never gave or took an excuse. Yes, I do see the difference now between me and other men. When a disaster happens, I act and they make excuses.[40]

And in a letter to Dr. J. Pattison Walker in 1864 concerning his pioneering work in sanitary reform in India, she challenged him:

You will have much opposition to encounter. But great works do not prosper without great opposition.[41]

Writing to her father on June 13, 1868, Florence expressed the burden of leadership in a manner with which most of us can identify.

And as for myself, I am so weary & heavy laden that, if the next existence for me were that of an owl, so that I could live for 100 years at rest, without any men throwing their business upon me which they ought to do themselves, I should be glad.[42]

Finally, in one of her last letters to the probationers and nurses of St. Thomas Hospital in 1881, she spoke of leadership thusly:

We need to remember that we come to learn, to be taught. Hence we come to obey. No one ever was able to govern who was not able to obey. No one ever was able to teach who was not able to learn. The best scholars make the best teachers—those who obey best the best rulers. We all have to obey as well as to command all our lives.[43]

Job Security (or insecurity, as the case

may be) was a concept that Florence understood to be a part of leadership and management. Today, we sometimes talk about how patient care administrators often feel a sense of playing "you bet your job" as they take risky actions throughout their careers. Florence was not immune to those feelings. While in Scutari, she wrote to her uncle, Sam Smith, on March 6, 1856:

am very anxious to correct a false impression, which seems to exist in your mind, that I have had a steady & consistent support from the War Office—that, such being the case, I kick against every prick—& am unduly impatient of opposition, inevitable in my or any situation, to my work.

The facts are exactly the reverse. I have never chosen to trouble the W.O. |war office| with my difficulties, because it has given me so feeble & treacherous a support that I have always expected to hear it say, 'Could we not shelve Miss N.? We dare say she does a great deal of good. But she quarrels with authorities & we can't have that'.[44]

Later in the same year after she left the Crimea, she wrote to Col. J. H. Lefroy (August 25, 1856), asking his advice on how she might best position herself to continue working with the military so she could

uggest reforms not within my power or province to execute.

Now, should I not cut myself off from all chance of ever obtaining employment in the Military Hospitals by suggesting the necessity of any great reform to my Magnates three _now_? It is certain that I should, were any of the Medical Magnates of the Army to have a scent of it?

Would it not be better for me to ask humbly & directly for a Female Nursing Department in the Army Hospitals, which I have little doubt the Queen would grant, without making myself more obnoxious than I am—or should I state boldly the whole case at first?[45]

Florence clearly thought that taking risks was a necessary part of the job, and in _Suggestions for Thought_, she stated her opinion of mistakes.

God's plan is that we make mistakes; in them I will try to learn God's purpose.[46]

Florence also spoke frequently about how to be a success as a leader. Among her most noteworthy suggestions were:

ever to know that you are beaten is the way to victory.[47]

It is a noble calling, the calling of Nurses but it depends on you Nurses to make it noble.[48]

I have never felt inclined to say 'resign yourself' but, overcome.[49]

We should strive for what we can best do and what is most attractive & thereby find our duty.[50]

Dare to stand alone.[51]

To a discontented nurse, she once wrote:

Do you think I should have succeeded in doing anything if I *had kicked and resisted and resented? Is it our Master's command? Is it even common sense? I have been even shut out of hospitals into which I had been ordered to go by the Commander-in-Chief— obliged to stand outside the door in the snow till night—been refused rations for as much as 10 days at a time for the nurses I had brought by superior command. And I have been as good friends the day after with the officials who did these things—have resolutely ignored these things <u>for the sake of the work</u>.*[52]

Florence saw what it would take for women to succeed in a "man's world" long before many feminists did.

would say of all young ladies who are called to any particular vocation, qualify yourselves for it as a man does his work. Don't think you can undertake it otherwise. Submit yourselves to the rules of business as men do, by which alone you can make God's business succeed. Three-fourths of the whole mischief

*in women's lives arises from their
excepting themselves from the rules of
training considered needful for men.*[53]

Florence's bigger aim was for people to
forget which sex should do what and just
have everyone, male or female, contribute
as best they could in whatever way they
could. In her final note in *Notes on Nursing*, she said:

would earnestly ask my sisters to
keep clear of both the jargons now
current everywhere (for they <u>are</u> equally
jargous); of the jargon, namely, about the
"rights" of women, which urges women to
do all that men do, including the medical
and other professions, merely because men
do it, and without regard to whether it <u>is</u>
the best that women can do; and of the
jargon which urges women to do nothing
that men do, merely because they are
women, and should be "recalled to a sense
of their duty as women," and because
"this is women's work," and "that is
men's," and "these are things which

women should not do," which is all
assertion, and nothing more. Surely
woman should bring the best she has,
<u>whatever</u> that is, to the work of God's
world, without attending to either of these
cries. For what are they, both of them, the
one <u>just</u> as much as the other, but
listening to the "what people will say," to
opinion, to the "voices from without?"
And as a wise man has said, no one has
ever done anything great or useful by
listening to the voices from without.

You do not want the effect of your good
things to be, "How wonderful for a
<u>woman</u>!" nor would you be deterred from
good things by hearing it said, "Yes, but
she ought not to have done this, because
it is not suitable for a woman." But you
want to do the thing that is good, whether
it is "suitable for a woman" or not.

It does not make a thing good, that it
is remarkable that a woman should have
been able to do it. Neither does it make a
thing bad, which would have been good
had a man done it, that it has been done
by a woman.

Oh, leave these jargons, and go your
way straight to God's work, in simplicity
and singleness of heart.[54]

In an address to the students and nurses
of St. Thomas in 1874, Florence summarized her description of a nursing leader.

She must have an iron sense of
truth and right for herself and
others, and a golden sense of love and
charity for them.
When a future Sister unites the power
of command with the power of thought
and love, when she can raise herself and
others above the commonplaces of a
common self without disregarding any of
our common feelings, when she can plan
and effect any reforms wanted step-by-step,
without trying to precipitate them into a
single year or month, neither hasting nor
delaying: That is indeed a "Sister."[55]

Everything which succeeds is not the production of a scheme, of rules and of regulations made beforehand, but of a mind observing and adapting itself to wants and needs.

Negotiation

Florence was an excellent negotiator. One thing she clearly believed in was the power to negotiate before you take the job. Before accepting the position at Upper Harley Street, she negotiated for changes in the nursing arrangements and mechanical improvements, which saved the nursing staff time and energy, and, in fact, could be seen as a forerunner of the patient-focused systems being implemented today to help the nurse stay near the bedside. Patient bells were redesigned to ring by the nurses' room and to designate which patient had rung. A tray hoist was built to save time when serving meals and hot water was piped up to the floors so the nurses no longer had to carry it. As Florence noted to Lady Charlotte Canning, a member of the Ladies' Committee, which oversaw the Harley Street establishment, in a letter on June 5, 1853:

The nurse should _never_ be obliged to quit her 'floor,' except for her own

dinner & supper, & her patients' dinner
& supper—(and even the latter might be
avoided by the windless we have talked
about). Without a system of this kind, the
nurse is converted to a pair of legs.[56]

Florence used timing for negotiations in making the best of a "honeymoon" period after she had just arrived in a job. Less than a week after she took her position at Upper Harley Street, she challenged the admission policies of the facility and won, at least technically. Prior to her arrival, no Catholic or Jewish person could be admitted. Florence said she would admit them or resign. The governing committee changed the policy, although there is no subsequent record of a Catholic or Jewish person asking for admission. Florence also replaced the matron, created a new housekeeper position, and replaced the chaplain with a chaplain of her choice. When the house surgeon resigned, she took a leading role in selecting his replacement and in redefining his duties, though neither was within the province of her position. Finally, before her "honeymoon" was over, she insisted on starting to make rounds with the doctors.

She advised her colleagues to follow the same approach when negotiating positions. In September, 1884, she wrote to Mary Ann Everett Green concerning a Headmistress position Mrs. Green was considering at Girton:

Y ou should not undertake this most important & most difficult post without making a very clear statement to the Committee of the conditions (not, of course, using this word) under which you could alone accept it. This must be done if only in self-defense, because there is apparently no official definition of your position and duties . . . It could mean nothing but disaster for you & _for Girton_, & vexation for every one concerned; that you should accept the position & find it untenable by reason of conditions imposed upon you . . . Your friends could never advise you to accept a position which the world outside regards as one of responsibility & trust, when it is

really one in which there is no trust, &
in which therefore there can be no
responsibility in the true sense.[57]

The following month, Florence wrote
Mrs. Green two other letters, one about
the need for Mrs. Green to make her qual-
ifications known to the interview committee and the other about material Mrs.
Green should send the committee. She
suggested that Mrs. Green write a statement of her views on education in general,
but cautioned her not to volunteer information on her position on female education, which Florence thought the interview
committee might not be ready to accept.

Is not any general exposition of
your ideas as to female education
. . . <u>unless asked for by the
Committee</u>—simply enlarging the area of
attack,—without, I should fancy, doing
the cause any kind of good?
. . . You should act strictly on defensive,
stipulating for or explaining <u>such things
as you would feel were absolutely essential
to your acceptance of the post</u>, but no

others. If they could all go into one side of a sheet of note paper, so much the better.[58]

No system can endure that does not march.

Organizational Structure

Florence's thoughts on organizational structure have permeated many health care systems. The best summary of her thoughts on organizational structure is found in eight fundamental principles she developed for the Nightingale School and Home for Nurses at St. Thomas Hospital as identified by Barritt (1973):

1. Certain goals or tasks require organized group effort, hence organization.
2. Each organization has a primary purpose.
3. Financial control provides administrative control.
4. Leadership of an area requires expertise in that area.
5. Hierarchial leadership roles with clear lines of authority and responsibility are needed.
6. Groups require clearly defined rules and regulations to function together as an organization.

7. Decision-making must be based upon the use of accurate data.
8. Efficient use of manpower is essential to an organization.

Florence believed in a centralized authority. In a letter to Sidney Herbert written from Scutari in 1854, she said:

The grand administrative evil emanates from home—in the existence of a number of departments here, each with its centifugal & independent action, uncounteracted by any centipetal attraction—viz. a central authority capable of supervising & compelling combined effort for each object at a particular time.[59]

A House of Commons motion she drafted for Sir Harry Verney in 1865 included the following:

That inasmuch as the question of due care of the sick poor in the metropolis is neither one of local rating

*nor of local management but of
administration it is expedient that for the
sake of economy, uniformity and efficiency
that there should be one central and
responsible administration to undertake the
entire medical relief of the sick poor.*[60]

She expanded her thoughts on this further the following year in a letter to Edwin Chadwick:

*Uniformity of system in this manner
is absolutely necessary, in order
that the suffering poor should be properly
cared for, & in order that vacant beds &
places may be filled up, wherever space
exists.*

*All the Officers of these Infirmaries &
Asylums should be appointed by & should
be responsible to the central authority,
which is responsible to Parliament.*

*. . . Hence comes the necessity—
necessity as I think of it, of consolidating
the entire medical relief of the Metropolis
under one central management, which
would know where vacant beds are to be*

found, & so be able to distribute the sick as to use all the Establishments in the most economical way.

The administration of these Hospitals should be specially organized (as we have done in the Army.) The best Medical & Surgical advice should be found for them—and, as said above, there should be <u>direct responsibilities</u> in all Officers from below upwards, ending in Parliament.

. . . And as part of the general administration, a thoroughly efficient system of nursing Sick, Infirm, Incurables, Idiots, Insane, could be introduced.

. . . In practice, there should be consolidated & uniform administrative arrangements. Sickness is not <u>parochial;</u> it is general & humane.[61]

With regard to nursing, Florence was always clear that a nurse should head nursing, with the nursing leader reporting to the principal medical officer. When she decided to accept the position in the Crimea, one of her first priorities was to establish herself as the sole leader of nursing. Ultimately, when there were challenges to her leadership, she made it a matter for the

British cabinet and received official notification of her role.

In 1855 in Scutari, she wrote Lady Charlotte Canning in answer to Lady Charlotte's questions about how to structure civilian nursing. In reading this, one must remember that the Medical Chief was the head of the hospital as well as the head of medical care.

B ind the Superintendent by every tie of signed agreement & of honor to strict obedience to her Medical Chief. (I think it has been the defect at Koulale that this has not been done.) But let all his orders to the Nurses go through her. I mean, of course, not with regard to medical management of the Patients, but with regard to the placing & discipline of the Nurses. I have never had the slightest difficulty about this—the Medical Men always coming to me & saying, 'I want such & such assistance,'—and I always informing them of any exchange or removal of Nurses—& consulting them. But I would never have undertaken the Superintendency with that condition that the Nurses consider themselves 'under the

*direction of the Principal Medical Officer'.
I am under his direction. They are under
mine.*

*. . . Under these circumstances, therefore,
I must suggest that the Form of
Agreement should bind Nurses to
obedience to their Superintendent, the
Superintendent to the Principal Medical
Officer by another form signed by her.
But if the Medical Officer conveys his
orders, in the first place, to the Nurse, the
Superintendent can only interfere in the
second place. And there will be continued
quarrelling, which there has never been in
the hospitals under my charge.*[62]

Further along in the same letter, in a dis-
cussion about wages, she also noted that:

*he Nurses should be dependent on
the Superintendent for their
wages—entirely—as she alone can know
their deserts.*[63]

In a letter to her friend Mary Jones who
was the head of St. John's House, she
wrote in 1867:

he whole reform of nursing both at home and abroad has consisted of this: to take the power over nursing out of the hands of the men and to put it into the hands of one female trained head and make her responsible for everything (regarding internal management and discipline) being carried out.

. . . Usually it is the medical staff who have injudiciously interfered as "master." How much worse it is when it is the Chaplain . . . Don't let the Chaplain want to make himself matron. Don't let the Doctor make himself Head nurse.[64]

Despite her affinity for a central authority and sole leadership of nursing, Florence also was one of the first people in health care to recognize the need for and implement a form of participative management. It often surprises people to learn that in the Nightingale School, which was known for discipline, the probationers were actually invited to criticize their lectures, thereby initiating and participating in future changes.

There are two classes of people in the world—those who take the best and enjoy it and those who wish for something better and try to create it. The world needs the appreciation of the first and the discontent of the second.

Personnel Issues

Florence addressed a number of personnel-related issues, among them recruitment and retention, staffing, and staff training. She had some of the same problems with recruitment and retention we have today. In her first position at Upper Harley Street, almost her entire staff turned over in her first three months. Nurses were more scarce when she was recruiting for the Crimea than they are now. In fact, her recruiters had to offer almost double the normal salary for a nurse and promise a fifty percent raise after a year's good conduct!

Once she got her staff, her problems had only begun. She appears to have discovered early on that more staff didn't necessarily mean more work accomplished. As she and her charges were just getting settled in, she received word that another group of nurses and nuns had been recruited and were about to leave for Scutari. She immediately wrote Sidney Herbert and others to try and stop the second group from coming. In a letter to Herbert on December 10, 1854, she said:

With regard to receiving & employing a greater number of Sisters & Nurses, I went immediately . . . to consult Mr. Menzies, the principal Medical Officer, under whose orders I am.

He considers that as large are now employed in these Hospitals as can be usefully appropriated & as can be made consistent with morality & discipline. And the discipline of forty women, collected together for the first time, is no trifling matter—under these new & strange circumstances.

He considers that, if we were swamped with a number increased to sixty or seventy, good order would become impossible. And in all these views I so fully concur that I should resign my situation as impossible, were such circumstances forced upon me.

. . . Lastly, I have found from this last month's experience that, had we come out with twenty instead of forty, we should not *only have been less hampered with difficulties, but the work itself would have been actually better & more efficiently done. About ten of us have done <u>the whole work</u>. The others have only run between our feet & hindered us—& the difficulty of assigning them something to do without superintendence has been enormous. It is the difference between the old plough with the greatest amount of power & the greatest loss in its application—and the Gee-ho plough with reins—accomplishing twice the work with half the power & much more efficiently.*[65]

The next time you're in a staffing crunch, you might also take heart in knowing that the nurse staffing ratio Florence wanted was 20:3,000, rather than the 40:3,000 she had or the 70:3,000 she would have if the new group came out (no, the numbers are not a typographical error!).

Florence began to identify early what she wanted to see in a nurse and what she wanted them to do. In *Notes on Nursing* she said:

I am far from wishing nurses to scour. It is a waste of power. But I do say that these women had the true nurse calling—the good of their sick first, and second only the consideration what it was their "place" to do—and that women who wait for the housemaid to do this, or the charwoman to do that, when their patients are suffering, have not the _making_ of a nurse in them.[66]

And in her 1875 address to the nurses and students of St. Thomas:

A woman who takes a sentimental view of Nursing (which she calls "ministering," as if she were an angel), is of course worse than useless. A woman possessed with the idea that she is making a sacrifice will never do; and a woman who thinks any kind of Nursing work "beneath a Nurse" will simply be in the way.[67]

Finally, in a letter to Colonel Loyd Lindsey that was read to a public meeting where the group that was later to become the British Red Cross Aid Society was formed and was then printed in the *London Times*, she expressed her respect for hospital nurses:

> *f there is any nonsense in people's ideas of what hospital nursing is, one day of real duty will root it out. There are things to be done and seen which at once separate the true metal from the tinkling brass both among men and women.*[68]

In 1893, in a paper presented to the congress on hospitals, dispensaries, and nursing which was part of the World's Fair in Chicago, Florence defined the role of nursing by describing sickness and health.

> *ickness or disease is nature's way of getting rid of the effects of conditions which have interfered with health. It is nature's attempt to cure. We have to help her. Diseases are, practically speaking, adjectives, not noun substances.*

What is health? Health is not only to be well, but to be able to use well every power we have. What is nursing? Both kinds of nursing are to put us in the best possible conditions for nature to restore or to preserve health, to prevent or cure disease or injury. Upon nursing proper, under scientific heads, physicians, or surgeons must depend partly, perhaps mainly, whether nature succeeds or fails in her attempts to cure by sickness. Nursing proper is therefore to help the patient suffering from disease to live, just as health nursing is to keep or put the constitution of the healthy child or human being in such a state as to have no disease.[69]

Among her problems with staff nurses (even then) was adherence to the dress code. In a letter to Dr. William Bowman on November 14, 1854, she quoted a "speech" made by one of her nurses: "I came out Ma'am, prepared to submit to every thing—to be put upon in every way—but there are some things, Ma'am, one can't submit to—There is caps, Ma'am, that suits one face, and some that suits another, and if I'd known, Ma'am, about the caps, great as was my desire to come out to nurse at Scutari, I wouldn't have come, Ma'am." To Florence's credit, the nurse did not leave because of the caps. In fact, she stayed with Florence for the duration of the war.

Florence believed that one of her main jobs was taking care of her staff. As noted earlier, she demanded and received improvements for the nursing staff before she accepted her position at Upper Harley Street. When she set off for the Crimea, she was told that everything that she and her staff needed would be there. It wasn't, but Florence made sure that she found ways to provide food and clothing for her nurses.

She thought time away from the job was important:

All nurses must have holidays . . . a month's regular holiday in the year is not too much . . . if they are to maintain vigor of body and mind, and not wear out prematurely.[70]

For patient care administrators, her advice was for us:

Always to take your exercise time out of doors, your monthly day off, and your annual holiday.[71]

She respected the older nurse as well as the younger. In a letter to the nurses and probationers of St. Thomas Hospital in 1881, she said:

To our beginners good courage, to our dear old workers peace, fresh courage too, preserverance: for to persevere at the end is as difficult & needs yet better energy than to begin new work.[72]

To pit the medical school against the nurse-training school is to pit the hour hand against the minute hand.

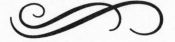

Physicians

Florence had her share of ups and downs with physicians, or "medical men" as she liked to call them. Some were among her best friends and some were among her worst enemies. An entire book was written on the subject in 1958 by Zachary Cope, entitled *Florence Nightingale and The Doctors*.

When Florence arrived in the Crimea, she met much resistance from the physicians, who made it clear that she and her nurses were not welcome. Her tactic was not to force her way in, but rather to not go into any ward or allow her nurses to go into any ward unless requested to do so by the medical director of that ward. Instead, she and her charges revamped the kitchens, cleaned up the hospital in general, carted away discarded body parts, and did anything else that would improve the sanitary or nutritional care given the patients. She was patient, knowing her time would come. It did. The influx of new patients rose to such an extreme that, within a very short time, she and her nurses were invited into the wards.

On November 14, 1854, less than two weeks after her arrival in Scutari, she wrote to Dr. William Bowman:

> We are very lucky in our medical heads. Two of them are brutes and four are angels—for this is a work which makes either angels or devils of men, and of women too. As for the assistants, they are all cubs, and will, while a man is breathing his last breath under the knife, lament the 'annoyance of being called up from their dinners by such a fresh influx of wounded.' But unlicked cubs grow up into good old bears, though I don't know how; for certain it is, the old bears are good.[73]

Florence clearly saw consistent, goal-directed work as the way to become accepted by the physicians. In her words to Sidney Herbert on December 15, 1854:

> I have toiled my way into the confidence of the Medical Men.[74]

As for working together, in another letter to Herbert two months later on February 12, 1855, she said:

What I *have done could not have been done had I not worked with the medical authorities, and not in rivalry of them.*[75]

It is in a letter to her Aunt Mai on October 19, 1855, that we see the ultimate attempt of the medical men to get rid of Florence by shipping her back to England without her knowledge. She had suffered from the fever while in Balaclava, and, having recovered enough to travel, was ready to return to Scutari. Two of the Army medical chiefs apparently had other plans.

It *is quite true that Drs. Hall & Hadley sent for a List of Vessels going home & chose one, the Jura, which was <u>NOT</u> going to stop at Scutari, <u>because</u> it was <u>not</u> going to stop at Scutari—& put me on board of her for England. And that Mr. Bracebridge &*

> Lord Ward took me out, at the risk of
> my life—to save my going to England,
> though unconscious at the time that it
> was <u>intended</u>.[76]

Florence and Dr. Hall had been locked in a long-term battle and would continue to be so for some time, but Florence kept some sense of humor about the relationship and continued to talk about Hall's good points as well as his bad. On November 17, 1855, she wrote to Elizabeth Herbert (Sidney's wife and Florence's friend):

> **D**r. Hall does not think it beneath
> him to broil me slowly upon the
> fire of my own Extra Diet kitchen and to
> give out that we are private adventurers
> and to be treated as such.
>   Remember, please, that this is quite
> private, that I do not wish to complain of
> Dr. Hall, who is an able & efficient officer
> in some ways—& that I think he has
> been justly provoked by Mr. Bracewell's
> 'Lecture" in the <u>Times</u> about English
> medical treatment—with which I utterly

dissent both as to its truth, & as to the
properiety of saying it, were it true.[77]

She was not enamored with the Army
physician corps in general and what they
had accomplished or more accurately not
accomplished, but she did not place the
largest part of the blame on the physicians
personally. As she wrote to Col. Lefroy on
June 9, 1856:

I *do not pretend to feel any respect*
for the Military Medical Profession
any more than for any other race of
slaves of whom they have all the vices &
all the virtues, but a strong compassion
and a burning desire to see them righted.
Of me they report things which they know
to be untrue, which they know that I
know that they know to be
untrue,—under cover of the confidential
report system which is practiced throughout
the Army and carried to its utmost
perfection by the present Inspector-General.[78]

Florence did have some clear feelings
about the interrelationship of nursing and

medicine. Cook (1913) quotes her as saying:

To pit the medical school against the nurse-training school is to pit the hour hand against the minute hand.[79]

The opinions of others concerning you depend, not at all, or very little, upon what <u>you</u> are, but upon what <u>they</u> are.

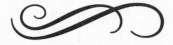

Power

Florence's ability to wield her own power as well as to wield the power of others for her causes was outstanding, especially in light of the societal positions of men and women at the time. After three months at Upper Harley Street, she wrote to her father:

he opinions of others concerning you depend, not at all, or very little, upon what <u>you</u> are, but upon what <u>they</u> are. Praise and blame are alike indifferent to me, as constituting an indication of what myself is, though very precious as the indication of the other's feelings.[80]

When her own power was not sufficient for her purposes she either went directly to more powerful persons and requested they speak for her or, especially in later years after her return from the Crimea, she did much of the background work for the powerful people. She began cultivating valuable relationships early in life, and by the time she left the Crimea, she had powerful relationships with the Queen, physicians, commissioners, members of the Cabinet, the media, and the general public as well.

In early 1855, she was very straightforward in a letter to Sidney Herbert:

> **Y**ou must write me, please, about the General Question (I am not now referring to the particular one of Nurses) a letter which I can show to Lord Wm. Paulet etc. besides the official one. The reason of this is that we find unwilling listeners, while you have willing ones—because what we have to say is troublesome.[81]

While in the Crimea, she also recognized the affect one person's or group's power can have on others. In a letter to Elizabeth Herbert in 1855, she said:

> **T**he real grievance against us is that we are independent of promotion & therefore of the displeasure of our

Chiefs—that we have no prospects to
injure—& that, altho subordinate to these
Medical Chiefs in office, we are superior to
them in influence & in the chance of
being heard at home. It is an anomalous
position. But so is war, to us English,
anomalous.[82]

Upon her return to England, she took
up the cause of sanitary reform for the
Army. After much lobbying and behind
the scenes activities, her commission for
Army sanitary reform was formed, com-
posed primarily of the people she had suggested and headed by her friend Sidney
Herbert, with a charge to do basically
what she had wanted it to do. She then
maneuvered to be requested to prepare a
confidential report for the commission on
the sanitary condition of the Army. Little
did they expect that they would receive an
830-page, well-organized report that not
only detailed (with graphs and charts) the
current condition of the Army, but also
proposed a totally new system that had
defined accountability and assigned tasks
down to the individual level.

Each person who received her report

also received individualized comments and suggestions. As the commission progressed, she supplied many of the commissioners with information about those appearing before it as well as questions they should ask.

Likewise, Florence played a major role in the Sanitary Commission on India. She collected data from every military station in India. When the Commission's 2,000-page report was completed, she abstracted it to twenty-three pages knowing that politicians and administrators especially would never read 2,000 pages. She even had a series of woodcuts by Hilary Bonham Carter included as illustrations to catch their attention. She sent copies of her abstract to virtually every influential person she knew. In a letter to Benjiman Jowett many years later in 1871, she explained her reasoning:

> There is no public opinion—it has to be created—as to not committing blunders for want of knowledge. Good intentions are not enough, it seems to be thought. Yet blunders, organized blunders, do more

mischief than crimes. Carelessness,
indifference, want of thought, when it is
organized indifference, . . . organized
carelessness is far more hurtful than even
actual sin, as we may have occasion every
day to find out.[83]

In another power move, she sent advance copies of the report to influential journalists. This was not the first or the last time she used this technique, having developed a long-term working relationship with several journalists, especially Harriett Martineau to whom she wrote on December 4, 1858:

shall be very grateful to you if you
will make use of my Report in the
way you mention. All <u>such</u> help is most
valuable to us. And, for the purpose of
putting you in possession of the exact
position in which our cause now stands, I
shall, if you will kindly allow me, send
you in a few days (i.e. as soon as it is
out) an answer which I have been forced
to make to anonymous attacks &
pamphlets, circulated without printer's

names, by traitors in our own camp.[84]

With regard to her behind the scenes work, she wrote to John Stuart Mill on August 11, 1867, in reply to his asking her to sit on the board of the new Women's Suffrage Society:

As to my being in the Society you mention, you know there is scarcely anything which, if you were to tell me that it is right politically, I would not do. But I have no time. It is 14 years this very day that I entered upon work which has never left me ten minutes leisure, not even to be ill. And I am obliged never to give my name where I cannot give my work. If you will not think me egotistical, I will say why I have kept off the stage of these things. In the years that I have passed in Government offices, I have never felt the want of a vote—because, if I had been a Borough returning two members to Parliament, I should have had less administrative influence. I entirely agree that women's political power should be direct and open. But I have thought that

I *could work better for others, even other women, off the stage than on it.*[85]

A major part of Florence's power came from her ability to identify stakeholders and their needs and desires. A prime example is contained in her letter to Edwin Chadwick on September 16, 1860:

ut above all I am anxious (and venture to suggest that it is most important) that the medical profession should not be indisposed to you, to the sanitary movement generally and to the Social Science Association in particular. Hitherto, to do them justice, I must say I think they behaved very well, and they have contributed their fair quota to the Social Science meetings. In particular forms of treatment they can (or the public think they can) give 'posers' to lay civilians 'interfering' in medicine. I am most anxious that this opposition should not be aroused. The sick are the most credulous of human beings. They will believe anything the 'Doctor' (whether allopathic, homopathic or hydropathic) says to them. For their sake let us be most careful to carry the 'Doctor' with us.[86]

She also talked about how to work with stakeholders.

The Supply and Demand principle, taken alone, is a fallacy. It leaves out altogether the most important element, viz. the state of public opinion at the time. You have to educate public opinion up to <u>wanting</u> a good article.[87]

*Patients won't wait to die, or better,
to be made to live, and operations
won't wait till I am less in a hurry.*

Time Management

Florence herself appeared to be an excellent time manager. Several of her biographers have gone so far as to suggest that her taking almost exclusively to her bed at age thirty-nine for the remainder of her life was her ultimate time management strategy. From that time forward, everyone (including kings, queens, and top government officials) came to her and on her schedule.

Florence thought that there was a need to be realistic about how much time a thing would take to be accomplished. A prime example was when she was being pressured to do something or at least to say what would be done with the Nightingale Fund (money that was being given to her by the public in appreciation for the work she had done, to be spent as she saw fit in developing nursing programs). While she was greatly touched by the gesture, she refused to just arbitrarily spend the money until she had the time to see how it would be best spent and to devote her own time to the projects on which it would be spent.

After a letter appeared in the *Times*, asking that she furnish a prospectus of what she would be doing with the money, she wrote to Sidney Herbert on January 6, 1856:

I think this is *perfectly reasonable, if I originally had asked for the money, which, of course, I did not. But to furnish a cut & dried Prospectus of my Plans, when I cannot look forward a month, much less a year, is what I would not if I could, & I could not if I would! I would not if I could because everything which succeeds is not the production of a Scheme, of Rules & Regulations made beforehand, but of a mind observing & adapting itself to wants & events. I could not if I would, because it is simply impossible to find,—time in the midst of one overpowering work to digest & concoct another—& if it could be done, it would be simply bad & to be hereafter altered or destroyed.*[88]

In a letter to C. H. Bracebridge later that same month, she also wrote:

In reply to your letter requesting me to give some sign as to what I wish to have done with the money— about to be raised under the name of the 'Nightingale Fund' & as to what purpose it is to be devoted to I can only say— 1. The people of England say to me by this Subscription—'We trust you—we wish you to do us a service'. No love or confidence can be shown to a human being better than this—and as such I accept it gratefully and hopefully. I hope I shall never decline any work God—& the people of England offer me. But 2. I have no plan at all, I am not new to these things. I am not without experience—and no fear presents itself more strongly to my mind, no certainty of failure more complete—than accompany the idea of beginning anything of the nature proposed to me—with a great demonstration—a vast preparation—a great man perhaps coming down to the Hospital—to give the first Cup of cold water'.

People's expectations are highly
wrought—they think some great thing will
be accomplished in six months—altho'
experience shows that it is essentially a
labor of centuries—they will be
disappointed to see no apparent great
change—and at the end of a twelvemonth
will feel as flat about it—as they do on a
wedding day, at three o'clock, after the
breakfast is over. But worse than this, the
fellow workers who would join me in a
work which began with excitement, public
demonstration, public popularity, w'd be
those whom vanity, frivolity, or the love of
excitement would bring—& these would,
least of all, bring about the wonderful
results w'ch the public w'd be
expecting—or rather the results w'd be
very 'wonderful' the other way. These are
not theories, but experience. And if I have
a plan in me, w'ch is not battered
out—by the perpetual 'wear & tear' of
mind & body—I am now undergoing—it
would be simply this—to take the poorest
& least organized Hospital in London, &

putting myself in there—see what I could do—not touching the 'Fund' perhaps for years—not till experience had shown how the Fund might be best available. This is not detracting from the value & importance of the 'Fund' to the work. It will be invaluable as occasion arises. I have hardly time to write this letter—much less to give the experience which would prove the deductions to be true.[89]

Time management to Florence also meant that there was a time to say "no" as well as a time to say "yes," although she said "no" much less often. In *Notes on Nursing*, she commented on the need to say "no" to constant interruptions.

I *have never known persons who exposed themselves for years to constant interruptions who did not muddle away their intellects by it at last.*[90]

Finally, Florence believed that nursing was a good apprenticeship for managing to get a lot of work done in a short period of time, regardless of how hectic the environment. In response to her long-time friend Benjiman Jowett, who had written to her concerned that she should slow down, she explained in 1865:

You are quite right in what you say of me. I mar the work of God by my impatience & discontent. I will try to take your advice. I have tried. But I am afraid it is too late. I lost my serenity some years ago—then I lost clearness of perception, so that sometimes I did not know whether I was doing right or wrong for two minutes together—the horrible loneliness—but I don't mean to waste your time. Only I would say that my life having been a fever, not even a fitful one, is not my own fault. Neck or nothing, has been all my public life. It has never been in my power to arrange my work. No more than I could help having to receive & provide for 4000 Patients in 17 days (in the Crimean War) and how easy that was compared to what has happened *since! Could I help—in the two R. Commissions I have served, in the 9 years I have served the W.O. exclusive of the Crimean War, my whole life being a hurry: if the thing were not done to the day, it would not be done at all. Nursing was a good apprenticeship.*

Patients won't wait to die, or better, to be made to live, and operations won't wait till I am less in a hurry.[91]

A Final Note from Florence

Let us be anxious to do well, not for selfish praise but to honour & advance the cause, the work we have taken up. Let us value our training not as it makes us cleverer or superior to others, but inasmuch as it enables us to be more useful & helpful to our fellow creatures, the sick, who most want our help. Let it be our ambition to be thorough good women, good nurses, and never let us be ashamed of the name of 'nurse.' [92]

References

1. Bishop, W.J. (1981). Florence Nightingale's message for today. In Herbert, R.G. (Ed.), *Florence Nightingale: Saint, Reformer, or Rebel?* (pp. 191-201). Malabar, Florida: Robert E. Krieger Publishing Company. (p. 200; 1893 Address to a congress on hospitals, dispensaries, and nursing at the World's Fair in Chicago).
2. Barritt, E.R. (1975). *Florence Nightingale: Her Wit and Wisdom*. Mount Vernon, New York: Peter Pauper Press. (p. 52).
3. Nightingale, F. (1914). *Florence Nightingale to Her Nurses: A Selection From Miss Nightingale's Addresses to Probationers and Nurses of the Nightingale School at St. Thomas's Hospital*. London: Macmillan & Co. (p. 5; May, 1872, Address).
4. Nightingale, F. (1914). *Florence Nightingale to Her Nurses: A Selection From Miss Nightingale's Addresses to Probationers and Nurses of the Nightingale School at St. Thomas's Hospital*. London: Macmillan & Co. (p. 1; May, 1872, Address).
5. Barritt, E.R. (1975). *Florence Nightingale: Her Wit and Wisdom*. Mount Vernon, New York: Peter Pauper Press. (p. 14).
6. Barritt, E.R. (1975). *Florence Nightingale: Her Wit and Wisdom*. Mount Vernon, New York: Peter Pauper Press. (p. 38).
7. British Library Additional Manuscripts 43393: f209 (January 6, 1956, to Sidney Herbert).

8. British Library Additional Manuscripts 43393: ff45–50 (December 25, 1854, to Sidney Herbert).

9. British Library Additional Manuscripts 43402: ff178–187 (1857, Private Note).

10. British Library Additional Manuscripts 45790: ff152–156 (December 3, 1853, to Florence's father, W.E. Nightingale).

11. British Library Additional Manuscripts 45790: ff152–156 (December 3, 1853, to Florence's father, W.E. Nightingale).

12. Nightingale, F. (1914). *Florence Nightingale to Her Nurses: A Selection From Miss Nightingale's Addresses to Probationers and Nurses of the Nightingale School at St. Thomas's Hospital*. London: Macmillan & Co. (p. 10; May, 1872, Address).

13. Vicinus, M. & Nergaard, B. (Eds.) (1990). *Ever Yours, Florence Nightingale: Selected Letters*. Cambridge, Mass.: Harvard University Press. (p. 385, May 6, 1881, Address).

14. Verney, H. (Ed.) (1970). *Florence Nightingale at Harley Street: Her Reports to the Governors of Her Nursing Home, 1853–4*. London: J.M. Dent & Sons Ltd. (p. 15; February 20, 1854, Report to the Ladies' Committee at Upper Harley Street).

15. Woodham-Smith, C. (1953). *Lady-In-Chief: The Story of Florence Nightingale*. London: Methuen & Co. Ltd. (p. 121; 1854, to Florence's father).

16. Nightingale, F. (1863). *Notes on Hospitals*. London: Longman, Green, Longman, Roberts & Green. (p. 107).

17. Nightingale, F. (1863). *Notes on Hospitals*. London: Longman, Green, Longman, Roberts & Green. (Preface).

18. Nightingale, F. (1871). *Introductory Notes on Lying-In Institutions*. London: Longman, Green, and Co. (p. 73).

19. Bishop, W.J. (1981). Florence Nightingale's message for today. In Herbert, R.G. (Ed.), *Florence Nightingale: Saint, Reformer, or Rebel?* (pp. 191–201). Malabar, Florida: Robert E. Krieger Publishing Company. (p. 201; 1893 Address to a congress on hospitals, dispensaries, and nursing at the World's Fair in Chicago).

20. Nightingale, F. (1863). *Notes on Hospitals*. London: Longman, Green, Longman, Roberts & Green. (p. 49).

21. Nightingale, F. (1863). *Notes on Hospitals*. London: Longman, Green, Longman, Roberts & Green. (p. 91).

22. Thompson, J.D. (1981). The passionate humanist: From Nightingale to new nurse. In Herbert, R.G. (Ed.), *Florence Nightingale: Saint, Reformer, or Rebel?* (pp. 220–230). Malabar, Florida: Robert E. Krieger Publishing Company. (p. 226; 1860 Presentation to the International Statistical Conference).

23. Thompson, J.D. (1981). The passionate humanist: From Nightingale to new nurse. In Herbert, R.G. (Ed.), *Florence Nightingale: Saint, Reformer, or Rebel?* (pp. 220–230). Malabar, Florida: Robert E. Krieger Publishing Company. (p. 226; 1860 Presentation to the International Statistical Conference).

24. Thompson, J.D. (1981). The passionate humanist: From Nightingale to new nurse. In Herbert, R.G. (Ed.), *Florence Nightingale: Saint, Reformer,*

or Rebel? (pp. 220–230). Malabar, Florida: Robert E. Krieger Publishing Company. (pp. 226–227; 1860 Presentation to the International Statistical Conference).

25. Nightingale, F. (1863). *Notes on Hospitals*. London: Longman, Green, Longman, Roberts & Green. (pp. 2–5).
26. Nightingale, F. (1863). *Notes on Hospitals*. London: Longman, Green, Longman, Roberts & Green. (pp. 175–176).
27. Nightingale, F. (1914). *Florence Nightingale to Her Nurses: A Selection From Miss Nightingale's Addresses to Probationers and Nurses of the Nightingale School at St. Thomas's Hospital*. London: Macmillan & Co. (p. 49; May 23, 1873, Address).
28. Nightingale, F. (1914). *Florence Nightingale to Her Nurses: A Selection From Miss Nightingale's Addresses to Probationers and Nurses of the Nightingale School at St. Thomas's Hospital*. London: Macmillan & Co. (p. 90; May 26, 1875, Address).
29. Woodham-Smith, C. (1953). *Lady-In-Chief: The Story of Florence Nightingale*. London: Methuen & Co. Ltd. (p. 121; 1854, to Florence's father).
30. Nightingale, F. (1859). *Notes on Nursing: What It Is and What It Is Not*. London: Harrison & Sons. (pp. 20–21).
31. Nightingale, F. (1859). *Notes on Nursing: What It Is and What It Is Not*. London: Harrison & Sons. (p. 23).
32. Nightingale, F. (1859). *Notes on Nursing: What It Is and What It Is Not*. London: Harrison & Sons. (p. 24).

33. Nightingale, F. (1859). *Notes on Nursing: What It Is and What It Is Not*. London: Harrison & Sons. (p. 24).
34. Nightingale, F. (1859). *Notes on Nursing: What It Is and What It Is Not*. London: Harrison & Sons. (p. 24).
35. Nightingale, F. (1859). *Notes on Nursing: What It Is and What It Is Not*. London: Harrison & Sons. (p. 25).
36. Nightingale, F. (1859). *Notes on Nursing: What It Is and What It Is Not*. London: Harrison & Sons. (pp. 16–17).
37. Nightingale, F. (1914). *Florence Nightingale to Her Nurses: A Selection From Miss Nightingale's Addresses to Probationers and Nurses of the Nightingale School at St. Thomas's Hospital*. London: Macmillan & Co. (pp. 12–14; May, 1872, Address).
38. Nightingale, F. (1914). *Florence Nightingale to Her Nurses: A Selection From Miss Nightingale's Addresses to Probationers and Nurses of the Nightingale School at St. Thomas's Hospital*. London: Macmillan & Co. (p. 16; May, 1872, Address).
39. Vicinus, M. & Nergaard, B. (Eds.) (1990). *Ever Yours, Florence Nightingale: Selected Letters*. Cambridge, Mass.: Harvard University Press. (pp. 91–92; December 5, 1854, to her family).
40. Cook, E. (1913). *The Life of Florence Nightingale: Volumes I & II*. London: Macmillan & Co., Ltd. (Vol I, p. 506; 1861, to Hilary Bonham Carter).
41. British Library Additional Manuscripts 45781: ff219–222 (June 3, 1864, to Dr. J. Pattison Walker).
42. Vicinus, M. & Nergaard, B. (Eds.) (1990). *Ever

Yours, Florence Nightingale: Selected Letters. Cambridge, Mass.: Harvard University Press. (p. 296; June 13, 1868, to her father).

43. Vicinus, M. & Nergaard, B. (Eds.) (1990). *Ever Yours, Florence Nightingale: Selected Letters*. Cambridge, Mass.: Harvard University Press. (p. 385; May 6, 1881, Address).

44. British Library Additional Manuscripts 45792: ff17–18 (March 6, 1856, to Sam Smith).

45. British Library Additional Manuscripts 43397: ff240–243 (August 25, 1856, to Col. J.H. Lefroy).

46. Nightingale, F. (1860). *Suggestions for Thought to the Searchers After Truth Among the Artisans of England*. London: Eyre & Spottiswoode. (p. 90).

47. Cook, E. (1913). *The Life of Florence Nightingale: Volumes I & II*. London: Macmillan & Co., Ltd. (Vol II, p. 273; 1877).

48. British Library Additional Manuscripts 45813: ff219–224 (August 4, 1896, to Julia Ann Elizabeth Roundell).

49. Goldsmith, M. (1937). *Florence Nightingale: The Woman and The Legend*. London: Hodder & Stroughten. (p. 74).

50. British Library Additional Manuscripts 45838: ff220 (Nightingale, F. (1851–52) *Suggestions For Thought* Draft).

51. Nightingale, F. (1914). *Florence Nightingale to Her Nurses: A Selection From Miss Nightingale's Addresses to Probationers and Nurses of the Nightingale School at St. Thomas's Hospital*. London: Macmillan & Co. (p. 126; April 28, 1876, Address).

52. Cook, E. (1913). *The Life of Florence Nightingale: Volumes I & II*. London: Macmillan & Co., Ltd. (Vol II, p. 195; April 22, 1869, to a discontented nurse).

53. Tooley, S.A. (1905). *The Life of Florence Nightingale*. London: S.H. Bousfield. (p. 48).

54. Nightingale, F. (1859). *Notes on Nursing: What It Is and What It Is Not*. London: Harrison & Sons. (p. 76).

55. Nightingale, F. (1914). *Florence Nightingale to Her Nurses: A Selection From Miss Nightingale's Addresses to Probationers and Nurses of the Nightingale School at St. Thomas's Hospital*. London: Macmillan & Co. (p. 82; July 23, 1874, Address).

56. British Library Additional Manuscripts 45796: ff39–42 (June 5, 1853, to Lady Charlotte Canning).

57. Monteiro, L.A. (1974). *Letters of Florence Nightingale in the History of Nursing Archive Special Collections, Boston University Libraries*. Boston: Boston University Muger Memorial Library Nursing Archive. (p. xviii).

58. Monteiro, L.A. (1974). *Letters of Florence Nightingale in the History of Nursing Archive Special Collections, Boston University Libraries*. Boston: Boston University Muger Memorial Library Nursing Archive. (p. 47).

59. British Library Additional Manuscripts 43393: ff22–32 (December 10, 1854, to Sidney Herbert).

60. British Library Additional Manuscripts 45799: ff119–121 (June, 1865).

61. British Library Additional Manuscripts 45771:

ff102–110 (July 9, 1866, to Edwin Chadwick).

62. Vicinus, M. & Nergaard, B. (Eds.) (1990). *Ever Yours, Florence Nightingale: Selected Letters*. Cambridge, Mass.: Harvard University Press. (pp. 121–127; September 9, 1855, to Lady Charlotte Canning).

63. Vicinus, M. & Nergaard, B. (Eds.) (1990). *Ever Yours, Florence Nightingale: Selected Letters*. Cambridge, Mass.: Harvard University Press. (pp. 121–127; September 9, 1855, to Lady Charlotte Canning).

64. Bullough, V., Bullough, B., & Stanton, M. (Eds.) (1990). *Florence Nightingale and Her Era: A Collection of New Scholarship*. New York: Garland Publishing Inc. (p. 177; 1867, to Mary Jones).

65. British Library Additional Manuscripts 43393: ff22–32 (December 10, 1854, to Sidney Herbert).

66. Nightingale, F. (1859). *Notes on Nursing: What It Is and What It Is Not*. London: Harrison & Sons. (p. 13).

67. Nightingale, F. (1914). *Florence Nightingale to Her Nurses: A Selection From Miss Nightingale's Addresses to Probationers and Nurses of the Nightingale School at St. Thomas's Hospital*. London: Macmillan & Co. (pp. 107–108; May 26, 1875, Address).

68. *London Times*, August 5, 1870, to Col. Loyd Lindsey.

69. Bishop, W.J. (1981). Florence Nightingale's message for today. In Hebert, R.G. (Ed.), *Florence Nightingale: Saint, Reformer, or Rebel?* (pp. 191–201). Malabar, Florida: Robert E. Krieger Publishing Company. (p. 200).

70. Barritt, E.R. (1975). *Florence Nightingale: Her Wit and Wisdom*. Mount Vernon, New York: Peter Pauper Press. (p. 21).

71. Nightingale, F. (1914). *Florence Nightingale to Her Nurses: A Selection From Miss Nightingale's Addresses to Probationers and Nurses of the Nightingale School at St. Thomas's Hospital*. London: Macmillan & Co. (pp. 77–78; July 23, 1874, Address).

72. Vicinus, M. & Nergaard, B. (Eds.) (1990). *Ever Yours, Florence Nightingale: Selected Letters*. Cambridge, Mass.: Harvard University Press. (p. 385; May 6, 1881, Address).

73. Goldie, S.M. (Ed.) (1987). *"I Have Done My Duty": Florence Nightingale in the Crimean War, 1854–56*. Iowa City: University of Iowa Press. (pp. 36–37; November 14, 1854, to Dr. William Bowman).

74. British Library Additional Manuscripts 43393: f34 (December 15, 1854, to Sidney Herbert).

75. British Library Additional Manuscripts 43393: f146 (February 12, 1855, to Sidney Herbert).

76. British Library Additional Manuscripts 45793: ff108–109 (October 19, 1855, to Florence's Aunt Mai Smith).

77. British Library Additional Manuscripts 43396: ff40–45 (November 17, 1855, to Elizabeth Herbert).

78. Goldie, S.M. (Ed.) (1987). *"I Have Done My Duty": Florence Nightingale in the Crimean War, 1854–56*. Iowa City: University of Iowa Press. (p. 75; June 9, 1856, to Col. J.H. Lefroy).

79. Cook, E. (1913). *The Life of Florence Nightingale:*

Volumes I & II. London: Macmillan & Co., Ltd. (Vol. II, p. 270).

80. British Library Additional Manuscripts 45790: ff152–156 (December 3, 1853, to Florence's father).

81. British Library Additional Manuscripts 43393: f154 (February 15, 1855, to Sidney Herbert).

82. British Library Additional Manuscripts 43396: ff40–45 (November 17, 1855, to Elizabeth Herbert).

83. British Library Additional Manuscripts 45783: f252 (August 8, 1871, to Benjiman Jowett).

84. British Library Additional Manuscripts 45788: ff5–8 (December 4, 1855, to Harriett Martineau).

85. British Library Additional Manuscripts 45787: ff38–42 (August 11, 1867, to John Stuart Mill).

86. Cope, Z. (1958). *Florence Nightingale and the Doctors*. Philadelphia: Lippincott. (p. 21; September 16, 1860, to Edwin Chadwick).

87. Cook, E. (1913). *The Life of Florence Nightingale: Volumes I & II*. London: Macmillan & Co., Ltd. (Vol. II, p. 269).

88. British Library Additional Manuscripts 43393: f209 (January 8, 1856, to Sidney Herbert).

89. British Library Additional Manuscripts 43397: ff179-182 (January 31, 1856, to C. H. Bracebridge).

90. Nightingale, F. (1859). *Notes on Nursing: What It Is and What It Is Not*. London: Harrison & Sons. (p. 29).

91. British Library Additional Manuscripts 45783: ff35–44 (July 12, 1855, to Benjiman Jowett).

92. Vicinus, M. & Nergaard, B. (Eds.) (1990). *Ever Yours, Florence Nightingale: Selected Letters*. Cambridge, Mass.: Harvard University Press. (p. 386; May 6, 1881, Address).

Bibliography

Andrews, M.R.S. (1929). *A Lost Commander*. Garden City, New York: Doubleday, Doran & Company, Inc.

Barritt, E.R. (1973). Florence Nightingale's Values and Modern Nursing Education. *Nursing Forum*, 12(1): 6–47.

Barritt, E.R. (1975). *Florence Nightingale: Her Wit and Wisdom*. Mount Vernon, New York: Peter Pauper Press.

Bullough, V., Bullough, B., & Stanton, M. (Eds.) (1990). *Florence Nightingale and Her Era: A Collection of New Scholarship*. New York: Garland Publishing Inc.

Cope, Z. (1958). *Florence Nightingale and the Doctors*. Philadelphia: Lippincott.

Cook, E. (1913). *The Life of Florence Nightingale: Volumes I & II*. London: Macmillan & Co., Ltd.

Goldie, S.M. (Ed.) (1987). *"I Have Done My Duty": Florence Nightingale in the Crimean War, 1854–56*. Iowa City: University of Iowa Press.

Goldsmith, M. (1937). *Florence Nightingale: The Woman and The Legend*. London: Hodder & Stroughten.

Herbert, R.G. (1981). *Florence Nightingale: Saint, Reformer, or Rebel?* Malabar, Florida: Robert E. Krieger Publishing Company.

Huxley, E. (1975). *Florence Nightingale*. New York: G.P. Putnam's Sons.

Monteiro, L.A. (1974). *Letters of Florence Nightingale in the History of Nursing Archive Special Collections, Boston University Libraries.* Boston: Boston University Muger Memorial Library Nursing Archive.

Nightingale, F. (1858). *Notes on Matters Affecting the Health, Efficiency, and Hospital Administration of the British Army Founded Chiefly on the Experience of the Late War. Presented by Request to the Secretary of State for War.* London: Harrison & Sons.

Nightingale, F. (1859). *Notes on Nursing: What It Is and What It Is Not.* London: Harrison & Sons.

Nightingale, F. (1860). *Suggestions for Thought to the Searchers After Truth Among the Artisans of England.* London: Eyre & Spottiswoode.

Nightingale, F. (1863). *Notes on Hospitals.* London: Longman, Green, Longman, Roberts & Green.

Nightingale, F. (1871). *Introductory Notes on Lying-In Institutions.* London: Longmans, Green, and Co.

Nightingale, F. (1914). *Florence Nightingale to Her Nurses: A Selection From Miss Nightingale's Addresses to Probationers and Nurses of the Ningtingale School at St. Thomas's Hospital.* London: Macmillan & Co.

Smith, F.B. (1982). *Florence Nightingale: Reputation and Power.* London: Croom Helm.

Tooley, S.A. (1910). *The Life of Florence Nightingale.* London: Cassell & Company Ltd.

Verney, H. (Ed.) (1970). *Florence Nightingale at Harley Street: Her Reports to the Governors of Her Nursing Home, 1853–4.* London: J.M. Dent & Sons Ltd.

Vicinus, M. & Nergaard, B. (Eds.) (1990). *Ever Yours, Florence Nightingale: Selected Letters.* Cambridge, Mass.: Harvard University Press.

Woodham-Smith, C. (1950). *Florence Nightingale: 1820–1910.* London: Constable & Co.

Woodham-Smith, C. (1953). *Lady-In-Chief: The Story of Florence Nightingale.* London: Methuen & Co. Ltd.